Nutrition-Focused
Physical Exam for Adults

AN ILLUSTRATED HANDBOOK, Second Edition

Nutrition-Focused Physical Exam for Adults

AN ILLUSTRATED HANDBOOK, Second Edition

Editor

Cindy Hamilton, MS, RD, LD, FAND
Senior Director
Center for Human Nutrition
Digestive Disease and Surgery Institute
Cleveland Clinic

Contributors

Andrea Jevenn, MEd, RD, LD, CNSC
Lead Dietitian
Nutrition Support Team
Center for Human Nutrition
Digestive Disease and Surgery Institute
Cleveland Clinic

Peggy Hipskind, MA, RD, LD
Lead Dietitian
Nutrition Therapy
Center for Human Nutrition
Digestive Disease and Surgery Institute
Cleveland Clinic

Marianne Galang, RD, CSO, LD
Advanced Practice I Dietitian
Nutrition Therapy
Center for Human Nutrition
Digestive Disease and Surgery Institute
Cleveland Clinic

Cassandra Pogatschnik, RD, LD, CNSC, CTTD
Advanced Practice I Dietitian
Center for Gut Rehabilitation and Transplantation
Center for Human Nutrition
Digestive Disease and Surgery Institute
Cleveland Clinic

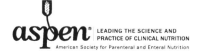

aspen® LEADING THE SCIENCE AND PRACTICE OF CLINICAL NUTRITION
American Society for Parenteral and Enteral Nutrition

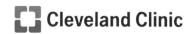

Cleveland Clinic

Published by ASPEN
8401 Colesville Road, Suite 510
Silver Spring, MD 20910
https://www.nutritioncare.org
aspen@nutritioncare.org

NOTE: This publication is designed to provide accurate authoritative information regarding the subject matter covered. It is sold with the understanding that the publisher is not engaged in rendering medical or other professional advice. Trademarked commercial product names are used only for education purposes and do not constitute endorsement by ASPEN.

This publication does not constitute medical or professional advice and should not be taken as such. Use of the information published herein is subject to the sole professional judgment of the attending health professional, whose judgment is the primary component of quality medical care. The information presented herein is not a substitute for the exercise of such judgment by the health professional.

ISBN: 978-1889622-50-7 (print)
ISBN: 978-1889622-51-4 (eBook)

Printed in the United States of America
10 9 8 7 6 5 4 3 2 1

CONTENTS

6 Functional Status 42

7 Micronutrient Status 46

PREFACE

The Cleveland Clinic Center for Human Nutrition (CHN) developed this illustrated handbook to assist clinicians with the nutrition assessment of their patients and to help discern the presence and degree of malnutrition. The Academy of Nutrition and Dietetics/American Society for Parenteral and Enteral Nutrition Consensus Statement and Characteristics for Identification of Malnutrition (2012) has been a catalyst for realizing the importance of incorporating a nutrition-focused physical exam (NFPE) as part of a comprehensive nutrition assessment. After the release of the consensus statement, the CHN developed a comprehensive training program—including online education modules and live patient simulations—to provide dietitians and students with a standardized approach for nutrition assessment.

The training program remains successful, however, it was evident that a learning tool with step-by-step instructions for performing an NFPE, along with visual aids demonstrating how to assess the physical findings, was needed. The result was the publication of the first edition of this handbook, containing photos, illustrations, and specific tips and techniques for performing the NFPE. This second edition contains new and enhanced photos and illustrations, information on examining and evaluating patients with obesity, tips for conducting telehealth appointments, and suggestions for electronic medical record documentation. We hope this handbook is a useful resource for clinicians and promotes confidence in performing an NFPE.

We would like to express our gratitude to ASPEN for their enthusiasm and willingness to collaborate with us to produce this valuable handbook. We appreciate the relationship cultivated with ASPEN over many years, which is one of collegiality and shared vision.

Cindy Hamilton, MS, RD, LD, FAND
Senior Director, Nutrition, Center for Human Nutrition, Cleveland Clinic

1

Introduction

Performing a nutrition-focused physical exam (NFPE) is a necessary component of a comprehensive assessment to determine a patient's nutrition status. Other components of the assessment, such as medical, surgical, social, and diet histories; laboratory data; and other pertinent tests are also required, but no one component can determine nutrition status.[1] The NFPE will help verify the physical changes to the body from undernutrition or overnutrition.

When determining patient nutrition status, the NFPE has not always been widely incorporated into the practice of many clinicians because of a lack of training or full understanding of its role as part of a comprehensive nutrition assessment. Many healthcare professionals incorporate a physical exam into their patient assessment, so it follows that the NFPE should be included to best understand an individual's nutrition status. It is particularly critical for hospitalized patients to have a full assessment. Full visualization, followed by examination inclusive of touch or palpation, is integral to determine body composition of fat and muscle, as well as the extent of fluid shifts. Additionally, the development of rashes; sores; or color changes to the skin, hair, nails, or oral cavity as a result of vitamin or mineral losses can be noted as an early sign of depletion. By incorporating all components of a nutrition assessment, the problem can be recognized, and a care plan can be appropriately designed.

In this handbook, contributors discuss the components of the NFPE and provide pictorial representations of various stages of muscle and fat depletion (ie, normal, mild, moderate, and severe), vitamin and mineral losses, and fluid balance. They provide techniques and tips for daily practice, along with useful tables and references. The Academy of Nutrition and Dietetics (Academy)/American Society for Parenteral and Enteral Nutrition (ASPEN) clinical characteristics and the influence of inflammation and functional status are also discussed.[2] This guide is intended to help clinicians develop their NFPE skills.

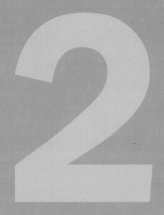

2

Preparation

FOR THE PHYSICAL EXAM

OVERVIEW

To conduct a comprehensive nutrition-focused physical exam (NFPE), the clinician must do some advanced preparation and incorporate a series of steps during the exam. Obtaining underlying information about patients will help clinicians create an informed context in which to attain additional or missing information and appropriately interpret the findings from a NFPE. Part of this assessment includes gathering information about nutrition intake and weight change using the Academy of Nutrition and Dietetics (Academy)/American Society for Parenteral and Enteral Nutrition (ASPEN) clinical characteristics (Table 2-1).[2]

TABLE 2-1. NUTRITION INTAKE AND WEIGHT-CHANGE ASSESSMENT: ACADEMY/ASPEN CLINICAL CHARACTERISTICS[2]

Malnutrition in the Context of Acute Illness or Injury		Malnutrition in the Context of Chronic Illness		Malnutrition in the Context of Social or Environmental Circumstances	
Moderate (Nonsevere)	Severe	Moderate (Nonsevere)	Severe	Moderate (Nonsevere)	Severe
% of estimated energy requirement		% of estimated energy requirement		% of estimated energy requirement	
<75% for >7 d	≤50% for ≥5 d	≤75% for ≥1 mo	<75% for ≥1 mo	<75% for ≥3 mo	≤50% for ≥1 mo

Food and nutrient intake. Malnutrition is the result of inadequate food and nutrient intake or assimilation; thus, recent intake compared with estimated requirements is a primary criterion defining malnutrition. The registered dietitian obtains food and nutrition history, estimates optimum energy needs, compares energy needs with estimates of energy consumed, and determines adequacy of intake as a percentage of estimated energy requirements over time.

Malnutrition in the Context of Acute Illness or Injury		Malnutrition in the Context of Chronic Illness		Malnutrition in the Context of Social or Environmental Circumstances	
Moderate (Nonsevere)	Severe	Moderate (Nonsevere)	Severe	Moderate (Nonsevere)	Severe
Time		Time		Time	
1%-2%: 1 wk 5%: 1 mo 7.5%: 3 mo	>2%: 1 wk >5%: 1 mo >7.5%: 3 mo	5%: 1 mo 7.5%: 3 mo 10%: 6 mo 20%: 1 y	>5%: 1 mo >7.5%: 3 mo >10%: 6 mo >20%: 1 y	5%: 1 mo 7.5%: 3 mo 10%: 6 mo 20%: 1 y	>5%: 1 mo >7.5%: 3 mo >10%: 6 mo >20%: 1 y

Weight loss. The registered dietitian evaluates weight in light of other medically relevant clinical findings, including the presence of underhydration or overhydration. The registered dietitian assesses weight change over time reported as a percentage of weight lost from baseline.

Systematic Approach to a Nutrition Assessment

Performing an NFPE is only one component of a comprehensive nutrition assessment. Clinicians often need to gather some baseline medical and nutrition-related details prior to the exam. Reviewing the medical record is an excellent starting point, and even though it is not a complete source of data, it certainly can be used to inform clinicians of gaps that need to be addressed during the interview and physical exam to ensure a thorough nutrition assessment is performed.

Gather as much of the following information as possible:

- **History and clinical diagnosis:** Reviewing the medical record for relevant past medical/surgical history, present illness, and clinical course will offer insight into the possible etiology and presence of malnutrition.[3] Some conditions affect the ability of patients to receive adequate nutrition and/or the ability to utilize nutrients, including specific disease states, surgical procedures, chemotherapy, previous hospitalizations, or severe trauma.[2,3] Acute conditions may be present with chronic conditions.[3] Refer to Section 3: Inflammation to direct further decision-making on this aspect.

- **Clinical signs and symptoms, vital signs:** These data may help identify factors preventing the adequacy of nutrition intake (eg, pain, nausea, vomiting, diarrhea, constipation) and characterize the presence and acuity of inflammation.[3]

- **Anthropometric data:** These data provide weight and weight history, allowing the clinician to consider the amount, percentage, and rate of change.[3]

- **Laboratory data:** Review data for evidence of hydration status, micronutrient abnormalities, inflammation, and protein-calorie malnutrition.[3,4]

- **Dietary data:** Use of the medical record to evaluate nutrition intake from all sources (ie, oral, enteral, and parenteral) may be highly subjective and is best corroborated against any further information obtained from the patient and/or caregiver(s). Evaluation of intake should be compared with the estimated needs of the individual as well as normal intake.[4] Identifying the degree of change is important for determining the severity of malnutrition.[2]

- **Functional status, as determined by strength and physical performance:** This is reviewed in comparison with normal activities and baseline strength.[5] Functional assessment must be viewed as changes occurring in relation to nutrition status. Changes in muscle wasting that make activities more difficult are considered to be nutrition-related functional changes.[5-7]

Interview Techniques and Tips

The next step of evaluation is to interview the patient. If the patient is unable to communicate, family and/or caregivers can help provide necessary information for the NFPE in addition to providing supportive data and dispelling conflicting information.

During the interview, maintaining focus on the severity and duration of nutrition-related issues is imperative for appropriate use of the Academy/ASPEN clinical characteristics.[2]

The goals when first approaching a patient to determine nutrition status include the following:

- Introduce yourself and explain the reason for your visit.

- Develop rapport.

- Gain the patient's consent to participate in the interview and physical exam.

- Ensure patient privacy throughout the process.

Interview questions should not be leading but should instead be open and probing to solicit impartial information. For example, it is not always possible to calculate the exact number of calories that someone has consumed over a particular amount of time. So, obtaining as much information on changes to eating patterns prior to (and during) periods of weight change may be helpful in estimating the percentage of needs that are being met. Examples of probing questions include

- Have you noticed a change in the amount that you eat at meals?

- When you are feeling well and eating normally, how is your eating different compared with now?

- How much are you eating compared with your normal amount?

- How often are you skipping meals?

- When was the last time you ate a meal that you would consider "normal"?

- How often does your infusion of enteral/parenteral nutrition meet the daily prescribed volume?

TIP When obtaining and sharing patient information, be sure to follow the Health Insurance Portability and Accountability Act guidelines for patient privacy.[8]

Physical Exam Techniques and Tips

Coordinate the entire assessment to include examination of muscle and fat stores, micronutrient deficiencies, and fluid accumulation. Physical findings should correlate with other clinical evidence already garnered from the medical record and during the interview with the patient and/or caregiver(s).

- Feedback from the patient is important, and it is most helpful to gather information while simultaneously performing the hands-on exam.[5] Frequently, patients will reveal more information in this manner than through the interview alone.[6]

- Prior to conducting the physical exam, explain the purpose relative to the patient's condition, such as introducing the exam as a tool to evaluate the baseline muscle and fat stores.

- Avoid terminology that may add to emotional distress. Clinicians should be sensitive to patients' feelings and avoid negatively describing abnormalities in body habitus (such as excess adiposity, extreme weight loss, or a suspected eating disorder) to prevent inducing further body-image sensitivities; instead, choose words that are more clinically or medically descriptive. For instance, when caring for a patient with cancer, they may be taken aback by a clinician saying, "You have lost so much muscle since I last saw you!" A better approach would be to gently educate the patient by saying, "It can be normal to see unintended declines in muscle and by understanding those losses with a thorough examination, we can develop a better treatment plan moving forward." Refrain from discussing any potential for recovery of weight, fat, and/or muscle, as this may not be possible. Do not make false reassurances about outcomes that may not be achievable.[9]

- Even if the patient does not consent to a physical exam, there are other methods to obtain information that can be used to determine an individual's nutrition status.[9] During an interview, the clinician can take note of exposed areas of the body (like the face, hands, and legs) and attempt to angle themselves so as to see these areas more closely or in different light. The clinician can also attempt to instruct the patient to pinch their skin under their own triceps or make an "OK sign" with their fingers. The clinician can ask more specific questions about muscle and fat changes to determine whether nutrition-related changes have occurred. These techniques can also be useful for telehealth appointments.

- This may seem like a time-consuming process, but with continued practice using a systematic approach, the clinician will become more efficient and find ways to incorporate personal touches to effectively assess patients.

Physical exam techniques consist of inspection, palpation, percussion, and auscultation. Because inspection and palpation are the main techniques used for the NFPE, only those concepts will be discussed here. Inspection is a visual technique that incorporates a broad observation of physical appearance, posture, color, texture, size, and symmetry. Palpation includes using the hands to examine for bulk, tone, texture, size, quality of volume/mass, swelling, symmetry, and temperature.[2,3]

Perform the exam at the initial visit and repeat during hospitalization to determine any notable changes indicative of a change in nutrition status.

1. Standard precautions

At the beginning and end of each patient encounter, it is important to diligently practice good hand hygiene to prevent the transmission of infections. This can be accomplished by washing hands with soap and water or by using an alcohol-based sanitizer. In situations when the clinician expects to encounter bodily fluids, skin wounds, or other infectious materials, additional personal protective equipment (PPE) including gloves, masks, isolation gowns, goggles, and face shields will be necessary. The extent

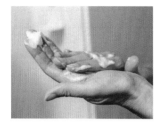

and type of PPE required is determined by the nature of the expected encounter. However, some infections will require clinicians to follow very specific PPE usage guidelines. Any time PPE is used, procedures for correct donning, doffing, and disposal of the equipment should also be performed.[10]

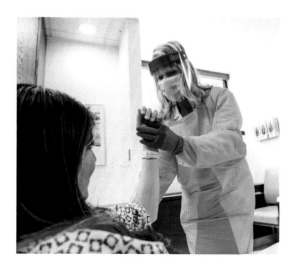

2. Start with a general visual survey

a. Pay attention to position/posture/physique.

  i. Is the patient sitting or lying in bed?

  ii. Can the patient maintain their posture?

  iii. Are there visible losses of muscle and/or fat?

  iv. Does the patient appear underweight?

  v. What medical equipment or devices might interfere with evaluating areas on the patient?

b. Make note of any obvious swelling, edema, or ascites.

  i. Could the presence of edema/ascites skew accurate interpretation of the patient's weight?

  ii. Are the legs elevated? For instance, upright positioning often shifts the location of peripheral edema to the regions of the body lowest to the ground (ie, ankles and feet), whereas supine positioning will relocate fluids to the thighs and sacral area.[11]

  iii. Alternately, does the patient appear overtly dehydrated?

c. Are there any signs of micronutrient deficiencies visible on the face, skin, hair, or nails?

3. Head-to-toe exam

a. Perform this exam using a combination of palpation and continued visual inspection.

b. Proper positioning is needed to perform an accurate and more reliable exam, assuming that the patient is able to adjust positioning without any medical or physical concerns (eg, fall risk, injury).

i. The clinician may need to ask the patient to change position (eg, sitting, standing, lying down).

ii. If the patient is bedbound, the clinician could try to have the patient roll onto one side or the other.

iii. If the patient is critically ill, the clinician will need to exercise care to perform an adequate exam without inadvertently disrupting tubes, drains, lines, and/or connections to life-support devices.

c. Move blankets, clothing, gowns, and compression stockings in a way that permits assessment of specific body areas but also assures patient dignity and privacy.

d. Take note of both the right and left sides of the body. Are changes unilateral or bilateral? Frequently, unilateral changes are not caused by nutrition issues.[9]

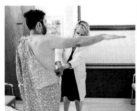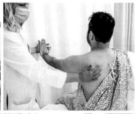
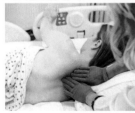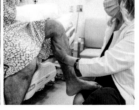

e. Communicate with the patient during the physical exam to help elicit additional information about specific areas being assessed while also minimizing assumptions. This type of communication is effective not only for interactions with patients who are hospitalized, but also for outpatient or telehealth visits.

i. Does your face appear thinner to you?

ii. Do your glasses or dentures fit differently?

iii. Are your clothes fitting differently?

iv. Do your [calves, shoulders, clavicle] appear different in any way?

v. Does your jewelry not fit well?

f. While assessing arms and legs, inquire about any physical signs of weakness that the patient may be experiencing.

i. Determine whether there is evidence that muscle weakness is related to nutrition status or whether the changes can be explained by other medical or physical circumstances.

ii. What is the patient's activity level now compared with previously? Inquire about types of activity (such as activities of daily living), the amount of activity in a day, and the time spent on additional activity (hours per day, days per week).

g. While assessing the head, neck, and orofacial areas, use a combination of interviewing and inspection techniques.

i. Are there any rashes or differences in hair, skin, or nails?

Nutrition-Focused Physical Exam for Adults, Second Edition

ii. Are there any chewing or swallowing difficulties? Taste changes?

iii. Does the patient report any mouth sores, tooth pain, or dentition changes that negatively impact food consumption?

Use of Inspection/Palpation for Specific Characteristics

1. Fluid and hydration status

a. **Inspection:** Assess the overt presence and general severity of edema, examine oral-cavity mucous membranes, and inspect skin for dryness.

b. **Palpation:** Assess the quality and severity of edema,[12] and check skin turgor and capillary nail refill.[13,14] Refer to Section 5: Assessment of Fluid Status, Tables 5-5 and 5-8 for further explanation of these techniques.

2. Muscle/fat

a. **Inspection:** Observe for texture and size; take note of symmetry and posture.

b. **Palpation:** Examine for bulk and tone of muscle and adequacy of fat stores. Refer to Section 4: Physical Exam of Subcutaneous Muscle and Fat Stores for details regarding each of these techniques.

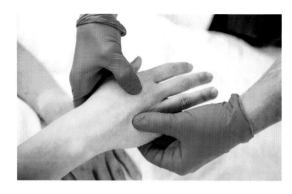

3. Micronutrients

a. **Skin**

i. Inspect for color, pigmentation, rashes, textures, dryness, and wounds.

ii. Palpate for temperature.

b. **Nails**

i. Inspect for color, texture, shape, and hygiene (consider beauty treatments, manicures).

ii. Palpate for capillary refill and frailty. See Section 7: Micronutrient Status, Table 7-2 for further explanation of these techniques.

c. **Hair**

i. Inspect for pigmentation/shine (consider chemical alteration) and distribution.

ii. Palpate for texture.

4. Orofacial/neck

a. **Eyes:** Inspect with penlight for color, abnormalities to appearance, and discharge. Refer to Section 7: Micronutrient Status, Table 7-4, for further explanation of this technique.

b. **Nose:** Inspect for color, texture, and discharge.

c. **Lips:** Inspect for cracks, lesions, color, and texture.

d. **Mouth/tongue:** Inspect with penlight for color, texture, hydration, swelling, lesions, dental caries, and erosions.

e. **Neck:** Inspect and palpate for swelling and symmetry.

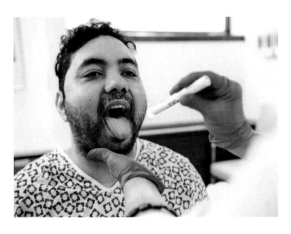
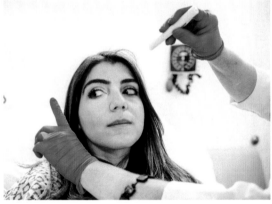

3

Inflammation

OVERVIEW

The Academy of Nutrition and Dietetics (Academy)/ American Society for Parenteral and Enteral Nutrition (ASPEN) clinical characteristics to identify malnutrition include determining the etiology of malnutrition. Etiology is determined by 2 main factors: the presence of inflammation related to the disease process causing a state of malnutrition and the length of time the disease/medical condition has been affecting the patient's nutrition status. To determine the etiology of malnutrition, the clinician needs to consider whether there is an inflammatory process present and, if so, to what intensity. Understanding individual patient situations in the context of different inflammatory processes will help more clearly define the varying effects and rate at which malnutrition may develop.[15] Several diagnoses can be categorized as an acute inflammatory condition or a chronic inflammatory condition (Table 3-1). When there is no inflammatory condition present, as with pure starvation, it can be categorized as a social/environmental/ behavioral cause of malnutrition (a semistarvation/starvation state).[16] Caution should be taken when deciding what is actually causing the malnutrition. For example, a patient with diabetes who lost their job several months ago may not be malnourished because of the diabetes but rather because of economic hardship, resulting in an inability to obtain food or medicine.

TABLE 3-1. COMMON DIAGNOSES ASSOCIATED WITH ETIOLOGY OF MALNUTRITION

Context of Acute Illness or Injury	Context of Chronic Illness	Context of Social or Environmental Circumstances
Heightened, High-Intensity Inflammatory State	Prolonged, Lower-Intensity Inflammatory State	No Signs of Inflammation
Abdominal abscess Acute respiratory distress syndrome Burns Trauma Major infection/sepsis Major surgery	Organ failure Cancer Cardiovascular disease Celiac disease Congestive heart failure Cystic fibrosis Cerebrovascular accident Chronic pancreatitis Diabetes Human immunodeficiency virus Lupus Obesity Pancreatic pseudocyst Rheumatoid arthritis Amyotrophic lateral sclerosis Muscular dystrophies	Achalasia Alcoholism Dementia Drug abuse Eating disorders Economic hardship Guillain-Barré syndrome Mental disorders Pain Sickle-cell anemia (pain)

This table is not intended to be a complete list of nutrition-related or nonnutrition-related etiologies.

Because determining the presence and degree of inflammation is not always straightforward, consider the following points for guidance:

- Acute inflammation signs and symptoms include swelling, erythema, hyperthermia, pain, marked C-reactive protein (CRP) elevation, and leukocytosis. Acute inflammation is a defense, clearance, adaptation, and repair response.[2]

- Chronic inflammatory markers may be the same as those with acute inflammation (eg, leukocytosis, fever, elevated CRP), but may appear to a lesser degree and over a prolonged period of time. Chronic illnesses or conditions may even lack the classic signs of the acute inflammatory process.[2,17] The purpose of a low-grade inflammatory response is restorative and is meant to achieve homeostasis.[17]

- Abnormal vital signs (Table 3-2), biochemical markers (Table 3-3), and imaging studies (Table 3-4) may indicate the presence of an inflammatory process, however, they may not be related to the patient's nutrition status and should be considered as supportive information when determining the etiology of malnutrition.

TABLE 3-2. MARKERS OF INFLAMMATION: VITAL SIGNS

Vital Sign Indicator	Abnormal	Special Considerations
Fevers	≥37.7 °C (99.9 °F)	May be masked by antipyretics (ie, salicylates, acetaminophen, NSAIDs)
Hypothermia	<35.0 °C (95.0 °F)	Rule out other causes
Pulse (heart rate)	>100 beats/min	May be masked by anti-arrhythmics (ie, amiodarone, disopyramide, quinidine)
Blood pressure[a]	<90 mm Hg >40 mm Hg drop from normal	Rule out other causes
Respiratory rate[a]	>20 breaths/min	Rule out other causes

NSAID, nonsteroidal anti-inflammatory drug.

[a] Based on systemic inflammatory response syndrome criteria for sepsis.

TABLE 3-3. MARKERS OF INFLAMMATION: BIOCHEMICAL MARKERS[18]

Biochemical Indicator	Normal[a]	Increased Levels	Decreased Levels
Albumin	3.5–5.0 g/dL	Dehydration	Inflammation Liver failure Nephrotic syndrome Fluid overload
Prealbumin	15–35 mg/dL	Fluid status change Chronic kidney disease Steroid use	Liver failure Inflammation
C-reactive protein	<1.0 mg/dL	Inflammation	N/A
Glucose, fasting or glucose, random	70–100 mg/dL <125 mg/dL	Diabetes Hyperthyroidism Pancreatic cancer Pancreatitis Trauma Stroke Heart attack Surgery Cushing's syndrome Infection Some medications	Reactive hypoglycemia Alcohol consumption Insulinoma Infection Organ failure

TABLE 3-3, continued

Biochemical Indicator	Normal[a]	Increased Levels	Decreased Levels
White blood cells, leukocytosis, or leukopenia	4500–10,000/mL	Anemia Some medications Smoking Infection Inflammatory diseases Leukemia Tissue damage	Sepsis Chemotherapy Infectious diseases Autoimmune diseases
Platelets, thrombocytosis, or thrombocytopenia	150,000–400,000/mL	Infection Kidney disorders Major surgery/trauma/burns Allergic reactions Cancer Heart attack Iron deficiency Hemolytic anemia Inflammatory diseases Pancreatitis	Leukemia Anemia Viral infections Chemotherapy Alcohol consumption Autoimmune diseases Some medications

Nitrogen balance	Positive	Negative:
		  Fasting
		  Illness
		  Infection
		  Stress	

Body fluid cultures	Negative	Positive: Infection	

N/A, not applicable.

This table is not intended to be a complete list of nutrition-related or nonnutrition-related laboratory values.

[a] These ranges vary from laboratory to laboratory.

TABLE 3-4. IMAGING STUDIES

Imaging Study Indicators	Acute Condition	Chronic Condition
Chest x-ray	Pneumonia Infiltrations	Scleroderma
Abdominal or pelvis x-ray	Abscess Acute pancreatitis Bowel obstruction	Chronic pancreatitis
Gastric emptying study, small-bowel follow-through	Bowel perforation Intestinal leak	Gastroparesis Dysmotility Fistulas Abscesses
Esophagogastroduodenoscopy or colonoscopy	Gastritis esophagitis Crohn disease or ulcerative colitis flare	Irritable bowel disease Radiation enteritis Strictures
Transesophageal echo	Endocarditis Vegetations	Congestive heart failure Heart-valve abnormalities

This table is not intended to be a complete list of conditions.

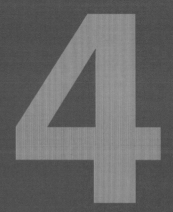

Physical Exam

OF SUBCUTANEOUS MUSCLE AND FAT STORES

OVERVIEW

One of the primary reasons to perform a nutrition-focused physical exam (NFPE) is to assess for the presence of and changes in muscle size and tone and fat mass, as part of defining malnutrition according to the Academy of Nutrition and Dietetics (Academy)/ American Society for Parenteral and Enteral Nutrition (ASPEN) clinical characteristics (Table 4-1).[2] Observation and palpation techniques of various parts of the body are used to determine muscle and fat stores, which is a subjective process.[6] Subjectivity of muscle and fat assessment among clinicians may be mitigated through training with experienced clinicians and repetitive practice using an NFPE.[6,19] Data about muscle and fat loss in patients from a physical exam have been shown to be readily available in the vast majority of hospitalized patients, including critically ill patients.[4,20]

Muscle wasting, or muscle atrophy, is a loss of bulk and tone that is detectable by palpation.[5,6] As stated by Puthucheary et al, "the loss of bulk and tone of muscle may not affect the person in a noninflammatory state, yet presenting in a more compromised position with decreased muscle mass promotes further reduction of muscle mass in critical illness."[6] This statement reinforces the importance of determining the etiology of malnutrition on the basis of inflammatory activity—not only the length of time the condition has been present. The moment of the assessment, along with the clinical condition, may affect a clinician's decision regarding the etiology and degree of malnutrition severity. This section will provide guidance about the specific locations to assess for muscle mass, muscle tone, and fat reserves and will also provide guidance for categorizing findings as normal, indicative of mild/moderate loss, or indicative of severe wasting.

TABLE 4-1. ACADEMY/ASPEN MALNUTRITION CLINICAL CHARACTERISTICS FOR MUSCLE AND FAT ASSESSMENT[2]

	Degree of Malnutrition	
	Moderate (Nonsevere)	Severe
Acute illness/injury (fat or muscle loss severity)	Mild	Moderate
Chronic illness (fat or muscle loss severity)	Mild	Severe
Social/environmental circumstance (fat or muscle loss severity)	Mild	Severe

Special Considerations: Obesity, Critical Illness, and Sarcopenia

Body composition, particularly the amount of lean and fat tissue, is a predictor of morbidity and mortality in critical illness.[21] When assessing for muscle and fat loss, there are certain circumstances or conditions that may interfere with a reliable physical exam.

Patients who have obesity may not readily exhibit visual signs of muscle and fat losses because excess adipose tissue limits observation and palpation of underlying muscle mass and tone. In addition, patients in the intensive care unit (ICU) may not be able to be fully examined because of limited patient participation; medical or hemodynamic instability; the presence of edema; or the presence of intravenous lines, drainage tubes, and other medical devices.[9]

The loss of muscle mass and subcutaneous fat can be evident within the first week of an ICU admission. It is therefore imperative to assess these patients early in the hospital stay and then serially.[22] Reexamination of ICU patients is important because changes (such as medical-device placement or removal and manifestation of edema) occur rapidly to reveal or hide areas that can be assessed for muscle and fat mass.[9] Additionally, increased patient mobility may allow for more areas to be examined that may not have been previously accessible to the clinician.

Per the European Society for Clinical Nutrition and Metabolism guidelines and definitions, sarcopenia is recognized as an inflammatory condition related to oxidative stress and is characterized by "progressive and generalized loss of skeletal muscle mass, strength and function (performance) with a consequent risk of adverse outcomes."[15] Sarcopenia has long been associated with the loss of muscle mass in the aging population, now recognized as primary sarcopenia. It is also a condition resulting from other factors, including disease-related, nutrition-related, and activity-related changes referred to as secondary sarcopenia.[15]

A considerable reduction in muscle mass is often accompanied by decreased muscle function, and it is suggested that when muscle mass cannot be assessed,

the muscle strength will provide supporting evidence.[23] There are no specialized criteria for classification and evaluation of sarcopenic obesity, and individuals with this condition are identified as a result of the evaluation of sarcopenia and obesity as separate components.[15]

Additional Tools for Body-Composition Assessment

Recent suggestions for body-composition assessment continue to recognize the use of dual-energy x-ray absorptiometry, bioelectrical impedance analysis, computed tomography, magnetic resonance imaging, and ultrasound, when available.[15,23] Images from these techniques are commonly obtained for analytical and diagnostic purposes, but can also be used to investigate lean soft tissue, an emerging trend to more clearly evaluate muscle mass, tone, and quality and fat as part of a nutrition assessment. Additionally, some clinical departments may have access to air-displacement plethysmography technology, dual-energy x-ray absorptiometry, and bioelectric impedance for a similar purpose. Assessing for loss of muscle and fat over time may prove beneficial to identifying changes that are otherwise limited to the physical examination process.[22] The expense of these technologies may be a limitation, and access to the necessary equipment may not always be available. The NFPE does not rely on expensive equipment and can be performed on most patients quickly and easily by trained clinicians.[20]

The measurement of muscle strength and function suggests the validated measurement of using handgrip strength as well as looking into the use of gait speed and chair standing tests as potential options for functional measurements.[15] Thus, inclusion of a physical exam, assessment of functional status, and determination of the severity of illness are all beneficial components when attempting to identify malnutrition or other nutrition-related derangements.[24]

Head-to-Toe Approach

The key to body composition assessment is being familiar with the regions where muscles and fat can be readily accessed and examined (Figures 4-1 and 4-2). A head-to-toe approach provides a systematic, organized-per-examination process for a thorough NFPE.[9] The upper body is more often used to help identify losses of fat and muscle, as it is typically less affected by edema, is more accessible to the clinician, and has been identified as a good reflection of overall muscle mass.[25] A thorough, bilateral review of the body during the physical exam is important for differentiating between nutrition-related wasting and wasting resulting from various diseases or deconditioned states. For instance, a patient who has a stroke or a broken leg may present with distinct variations in muscle tone on each side of the body. Nutrition-related muscle wasting is typically symmetrical, but other diseases also promote this type of wasting and should be ruled out during the nutrition assessment. To ensure the most accurate depiction of muscle and fat during the head-to-toe approach, patients need to be properly positioned.[9]

FIGURE 4-1. MUSCLE GROUPS FOR HEAD-TO-TOE ASSESSMENT

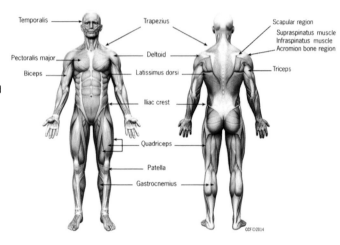

FIGURE 4-2a. EXAM AREAS: HEAD AND FACE (FAT AND MUSCLE)

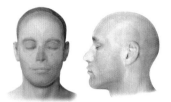

Normal

Orbital Region: Orbital fat pads
- Slightly bulged fat pads

Temple Region: Temporalis muscle
- Well-defined muscle, flat, or slight bulge

Mild to Moderate

Orbital Region: Orbital fat pads
- Slightly dark circles, somewhat hollow look

Temple Region: Temporalis muscle
- Slight depression

Severe

Orbital Region: Orbital fat pads
- Hollow look; depressions around eye; dark circles; loose, saggy skin

Temple Region: Temporalis muscle
- Deep hollowing/scooping, lacking muscle to the touch, facial bone structures very defined

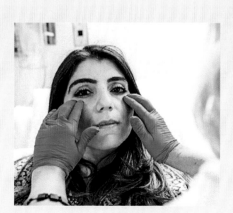 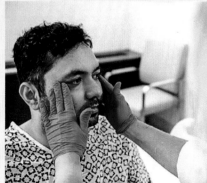

TIPS

Orbital Region: Orbital fat pads

Positioning: Frontal; lightly palpate above cheekbone

Temple Region: Temporalis muscle

Positioning: Frontal and side views

FIGURE 4-2b. EXAM AREAS: UPPER CHEST (MUSCLE)

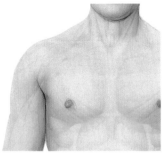 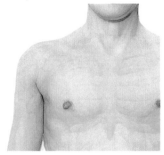 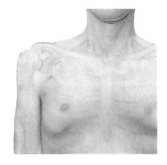

Normal

Clavicle Bone Region: Pectoralis major, deltoid, trapezius

- Well-defined muscle surrounding bone, clavicle bone typically not visible in males and may be slightly prominent in females

Acromion Bone Region: Deltoid

- Rounded curves at arms, shoulder, and neck

Mild to Moderate

Clavicle Bone Region: Pectoralis major, deltoid, trapezius

- More prominent clavicle bone, less prominent muscle when palpated

Acromion Bone Region: Deltoid

- Acromion process may slightly protrude

Severe

Clavicle Bone Region: Pectoralis major, deltoid, trapezius

- Protruding and prominent bone with low surrounding muscle mass when palpated

Acromion Bone Region: Deltoid

- Shoulder-to-arm joint looks square, bones more prominent, acromion process very prominent

TIPS

Clavicle Bone Region: Pectoralis major, deltoid, trapezius

Positioning: Upright and not hunched over

Acromion Bone Region: Deltoid

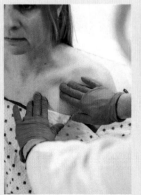 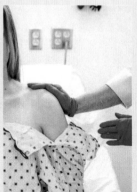 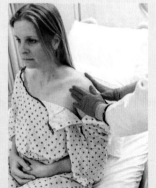

FIGURE 4-2c. EXAM AREAS: UPPER BACK (MUSCLE)

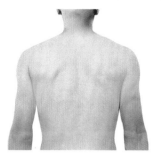 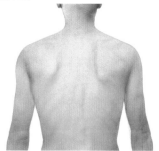 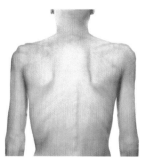

Normal

Scapular Bone Region: Trapezius, supraspinatus, infraspinatus

- Bones not prominent, no significant depressions

Mild to Moderate

Scapular Bone Region: Trapezius, supraspinatus, infraspinatus

- Mild depression around scapula or bone may slightly show

Severe

Scapular Bone Region: Trapezius, supraspinatus, infraspinatus

- Prominent, visible scapula bone; notable depressions between ribs, scapula, and/or shoulder/spine

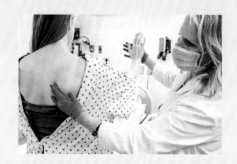

Positioning: Ask patient to extend arms out and push against solid object (clinician may use hand as support for patient to push against).

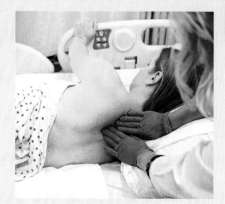

TIPS

If patient is unable to sit or stand, ask patient to roll to the side, extending arms as able, and push against a solid object.

FIGURE 4-2d. EXAM AREAS: MIDAXILLARY LINE (FAT)

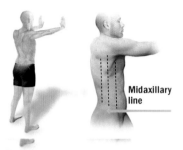
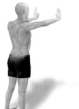
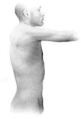

Normal

Thoracic and Lumbar Region: Ribs, lower back, midaxillary line at iliac crest

- Chest is full, ribs do not show, slight to no protrusion of the iliac crest

Mild to Moderate

Thoracic and Lumbar Region: Ribs, lower back, midaxillary line

- Ribs somewhat more apparent, depressions not very pronounced, iliac crest somewhat prominent

Severe

Thoracic and Lumbar Region: Ribs, lower back, midaxillary line

- Depression between ribs very apparent, iliac crest is very prominent

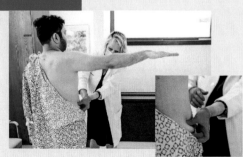

Positioning: Ask patient to extend arms out in front or out to sides of their body and push against solid object (clinician may use hand as support for patient to push against).

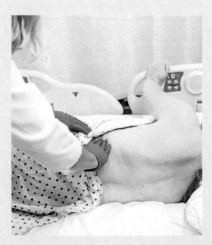

If unable to stand, patient may lie on their back (this may not be optimal to assess because of interfering factors in positioning).

FIGURE 4-2e. EXAM AREAS: ARMS (FAT)

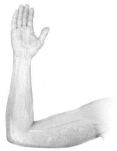
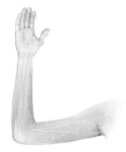
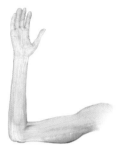

Normal

Upper Arm Region: Area under the triceps muscles
- Ample fat tissue obvious between folds of skin pinched between fingers

Mild to Moderate

Upper Arm Region: Area under the triceps muscles
- Some depth to pinch, not ample

Severe

Upper Arm Region: Area under the triceps muscles
- Very little space between folds, fingers practically touching

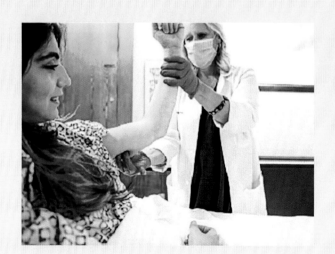

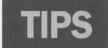
TIPS

Positioning: With arm bent at a 90° angle, use a gentle rolling motion between thumb and fingers down the triceps to separate muscle and assess fat.

Once fingers have pinched the area under the triceps, take note of the amount of fat between.

FIGURE 4-2f. EXAM AREAS: HANDS (MUSCLE)

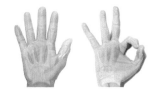

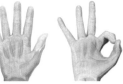

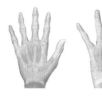

Normal

Palmar: Opponens pollicis, adductor pollicis, abductor pollicis, first dorsal interosseous manus

- Muscle bulges, could be flat in some well-nourished individuals

Mild to Moderate

Palmar: Opponens pollicis, adductor pollicis, abductor pollicis, first dorsal interosseous manus

- Slight depression

Severe

Palmar: Opponens pollicis, adductor pollicis, abductor pollicis, first dorsal interosseous manus

- Depressed areas, particularly between thumb and forefinger

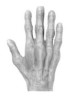

Dorsal: Dorsal interossei muscles, adductor muscles

- Flat/mild bulge between dorsal bones, bulging/flat muscle between index finger and thumb

Dorsal: Dorsal interossei muscles, adductor muscles

- Slight depression between dorsal bones

Dorsal: Dorsal interossei muscles, adductor muscles

- Depressed areas between dorsal bones, particularly between thumb and forefinger; bones prominent

TIPS

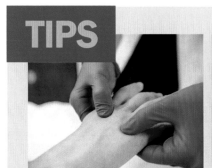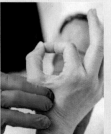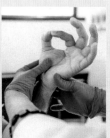

Positioning: Observe muscle pads where forefinger and thumb intersect while patient is making an "OK" sign. View and palpate dorsal and palmar sides of the hand.

FIGURE 4-2g. EXAM AREAS: LOWER EXTREMITIES (MUSCLE)

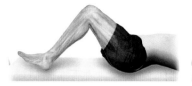 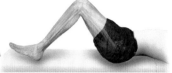 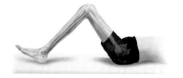

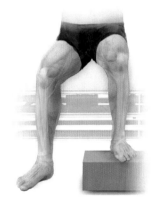 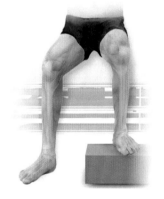 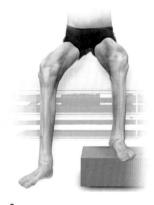

Normal

Anterior Thigh Region: Quadriceps
- Well rounded, well developed

Patellar Region: Quadriceps
- Muscles protrude, kneecap not prominent

Posterior Calf Region: Gastrocnemius
- Well-developed bulb of muscle

Mild to Moderate

Anterior Thigh Region: Quadriceps
- Mild depression on inner thigh

Patellar Region: Quadriceps
- Kneecap more prominent

Posterior Calf Region: Gastrocnemius
- Not well developed

Severe

Anterior Thigh Region: Quadriceps
- Depression/line on thigh, not well developed

Patellar Region: Quadriceps
- Kneecap prominent, little sign of muscle around knee

Posterior Calf Region: Gastrocnemius
- Thin, minimal to no muscle definition

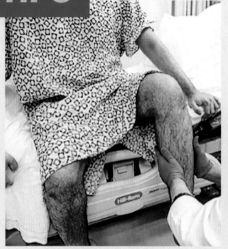

Positioning: Ask patient to sit up with leg propped up/bent at knee; grasp quadriceps/gastrocnemius muscles to distinguish between muscle and fat.

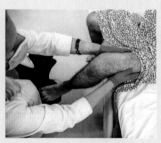

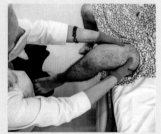

If patient is unable to sit up, have patient bend knee (while lying down) so that calf and quadriceps are lifted off the bed.

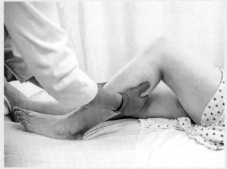

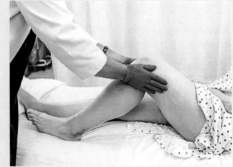

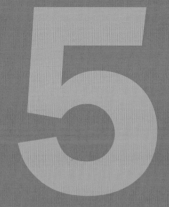

Assessment of Fluid Status

ACCUMULATION AND DEHYDRATION

OVERVIEW

Part of the nutrition-focused physical exam (NFPE) for diagnosing malnutrition includes the clinical evaluation of fluid status, specifically how it affects weight changes (Table 5-1).[2] Under ordinary circumstances, the human body is excellent at tightly regulating hydration and can easily adapt to fluid and electrolyte shifts while maintaining normal functions.[14] Healthy kidneys are able to maintain water and salt balance in the body, so unless there is an underlying systemic disorder, changes solely in water or salt intake should not cause edema.[26] Volume depletion, caused by interstitial and intravascular fluid movement into a third space, can present clinically as edema.[27]

Gross deficiency of protein for an extended period of time, the physiological response to refeeding syndrome, and some inflammatory responses to acute and chronic diseases can result in edema.[27] Fluid accumulation is rarely a direct manifestation of malnutrition but can present as weight gain, thereby concealing weight loss[2] as well as muscle and fat loss. On the other hand, dehydration can be a result of various medical conditions or not maintaining adequate nutrition and can manifest in an inaccurately low weight.[14] This section reviews physical exam techniques to assess a patient's fluid status as part of establishing a proper malnutrition diagnosis.

Fluid Accumulation/Edema

Edema is an excess of interstitial fluid accumulation that can be caused by a multitude of clinical conditions (Table 5-2) and medications (Table 5-3).[27] Clinically known as swelling, edema can be palpable and account for 10%–30% of body weight.[11,12] Systemic fluid retention may not clinically manifest until it accounts for at least 10% of body weight[26] or when interstitial fluid volume is increased by 2.5–3 L.[11,12] When the volume of edema is immense and can be readily observed, it is known as anasarca.[11] Extra fluid around the heart, fluid in the lungs,[27] small pockets of ascites, or hematomas might not be visible on examination and may be visible only on imaging studies. Therefore, a significant amount of fluid retention can be present without a patient actually appearing overtly edematous.[27] Less obvious clues might be present instead, such as ill-fitting shoes or rings, rapid weight increase, declining serum sodium levels, dyspnea, increased blood pressure, or distended neck veins.[11,27]

Fluid accumulation can be generalized or concentrated in one area (Table 5-4), chronic or acute in nature, unilateral or bilateral, or pitting or brawny. Distinction of these characteristics can help determine the etiology.[11,27] Peripheral edema gravitates to dependent areas of the body and is contingent on body positioning.[11,27] Observation of symptoms during a physical exam is equally as important as monitoring weight fluctuations to determine whether edema is worsening or improving.[11]

TABLE 5-1. ACADEMY/ASPEN FLUID ACCUMULATION CHARACTERISTICS THAT SUPPORT A MALNUTRITION DIAGNOSIS[2]

	Fluid Accumulation	
	Moderate (Nonsevere) Malnutrition	Severe Malnutrition
Acute illness/injury	Mild	Moderate to Severe
Chronic illness	Mild	Severe
Social/environmental circumstance	Mild	Severe

Impact of Edema on Nutrition

Based on the Academy of Nutrition and Dietetics (Academy)/American Society for Parenteral and Enteral Nutrition (ASPEN) consensus statement, fluid accumulation is one of the characteristics that supports a malnutrition diagnosis (Table 5-1).[5] Therefore, it is important to assess and monitor for changes (Tables 5-5 and 5-6). Nonetheless, caution should be exercised, as edema is rarely the direct result of malnutrition.[2,14] Edema can be a result of fluids shifting into the interstitial space from decreased capillary oncotic pressure caused by hypoalbuminemia, but hypoalbuminemia does not reliably correlate with malnutrition.[2,11] Edema explains rapid increases in weight, but it can also mask the severity of weight decline,[2] thereby impacting diagnostic accuracy of the presence and severity of malnutrition. Edema can also interfere with accurate examination of muscle and fat loss.[26]

TABLE 5-2. DIFFERENTIAL DIAGNOSIS OF EDEMA[11,14,27]

Clinical Presentation	Disease Association	Additional Considerations
Anasarca or generalized edema	Cardiovascular disease	Elevated venous jugular pressure, dyspnea
	Congestive heart failure	N/A
	Hepatic disease (cirrhosis)	Ascites; could also present as peripheral edema
	Renal disease	Usually chronic; presence of proteinuria, hypertension
	Nephrotic syndrome	N/A
	Glomerulonephritis	N/A
	Myxedema	Thickening of the skin; nonpitting, can be on lower extremities, hands, or face
Localized edema	Trauma	N/A
	Burns	N/A
	Angioedema	N/A
	Hives	N/A
	Skin infection	Erysipelas, cellulitis
Ascites	Cirrhosis	Anasarca; could also present as peripheral edema
	Hepatic veno-occlusive disease	N/A
	Malignancy	N/A
	Severe right-side heart failure	Anasarca; could also present as peripheral edema
Asymmetric/unilateral lower-extremity edema	Deep vein thrombosis	Primary concern; acute condition accompanied by pain, erythema, localized warmth
	Chronic venous insufficiency/disease	Peripheral, most common in legs (eg, after lymph-node dissection from cancer, causing nonpitting lymphedema)
	Muscle strain, tear, twist	Injury to the affected limb; acute condition
	Lymphedema	N/A
	Complex regional pain syndrome	N/A
	Compartment syndrome	N/A
	Pelvic neoplasms	N/A

TABLE 5-2, continued

Clinical Presentation	Disease Association	Additional Considerations
Bilateral lower-extremity edema	Chronic venous diseases	Most common
	Heart failure	Most common
	Pulmonary hypertension	Very common, but often overlooked
	Fluid overload	N/A
	Inflammation, sepsis	N/A
	Refeeding syndrome	May also present at generalized edema
	Beriberi	N/A
	Nephrotic syndrome	Peripheral and periorbital edema, occasionally with ascites
	Pregnancy	N/A
	Cirrhosis	Ascites can also be present
	Malnutrition/malabsorption	Uncommon, chronic edema; also generalized edema; protein losing enteropathy or changes in oncotic pressure from hypoalbuminemia
	Renal and liver disease	Uncommon; may also present at generalized edema
	Lymphedema	Not true "edema"
	Pretibial myxedema	Brawny, located on shins, not a true edema—rather a thickening of the dermis; may also involve toes/feet
Upper-extremity edema	Trauma	N/A
	Superficial thrombophlebitis	N/A
	Infection	N/A
	Arthritis	With inflammation
	Deep vein thrombosis	Especially if venous catheter is present
	Superior vena cava syndrome	N/A
	Lymphedema	Occurs gradually; in adults, can occur after radiation or surgery

N/A, not applicable.

List is not all-inclusive.

TABLE 5-3. MEDICATIONS KNOWN TO CAUSE EDEMA[11,26,27]

Drug Class	Medications
Antidepressants	Trazodone MAOIs (eg, isocarboxazid, phenelzine sulfate, tranylcypromine sulfate, selegiline)
Antihypertensives	Calcium channel blockers (eg, amlodipine, felodipine, nicardipine, diltiazem, verapamil) Beta-blockers (eg, propranolol, atenolol, labetalol, carvedilol, metoprolol) Vasodilators (eg, hydralazine, minoxidil, clonidine, methyldopa, guanethidine)
Hormones	Estrogen, progesterone, testosterone, corticosteroids, glucocorticoids, anabolic steroids, growth hormone
NSAIDs	Aspirin, ibuprofen, naproxen Cyclooxygenase-2 inhibitors (eg, valdecoxib, rofecoxib, celecoxib)
Thiazolidinediones	Rosiglitazone, pioglitazone
Anticonvulsants	Gabapentin, pregabalin
Antineoplastics/immunotherapies	Docetaxel Cisplatin Interleukin-2 Muromonab-CD3
Anti–Parkinson disease	Pramipexole, ropinirole
Others	Cyclosporine Proton Pump Inhibitors Tamoxifen

MAOI, monoamine oxidase inhibitor; NSAID, nonsteroidal anti-inflammatory drug.

List is not all-inclusive.

TABLE 5-4. TERMINOLOGY USED TO DESCRIBE EDEMA[11,27]

Term	Definition
Ascites	Accumulation of fluid in the abdomen causing distention; percussed shifting dullness and fluid wave
Anasarca	Massive, generalized, whole-body edema
Peripheral edema	Presence of excess interstitial fluid in tissue; pitting or nonpitting; characterized primarily by swollen lower extremities, with a tendency to accumulate in dependent areas (eg, thighs, sacrum with bed rest) and may cause ambulating difficulties
Pitting edema	Reflective of the movement of excess interstitial fluid; leaves indentation when at least 5 s of pressure is applied to edematous area
Nonpitting edema or brawny edema	No indentation is created after pressure is applied to the edematous area, characterized by thickening, dark color, dry/scaly patches, induration, and liposclerosis

TIPS

Assessing the quality of edema with palpation

Peripheral edema classification is subjective. Despite its subjectivity, use of a schematic can assist with recording changes in edema over time.[11,14,26]

1. Locate an area of the lower extremities where the skin overlies a bone, such as the shin, malleolus, or dorsum of the foot.

2. Using the pad of your finger or thumb, press down on the skin with moderate pressure for at least 5 seconds.

3. Lift finger from skin and observe indentation to determine severity.

   a. If indentation appears after pressure is applied, how deep is it?

   b. How much time passes until the area refills with fluid?

   c. How far up the leg can the edema be appreciated?

Remember, brawny edema will not leave an indentation, so use of the grading scale would not be appropriate.

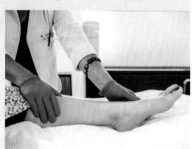

TABLE 5-5. GRADING OF PITTING EDEMA[14]

No Edema	1+ Edema	2+ Edema	3+ Edema	4+ Edema
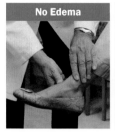	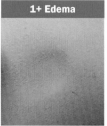	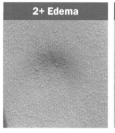	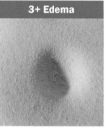	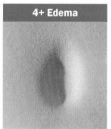

Grade		Method 1	Method 2	Method 3
No Edema		No impression or distortion observed, bone structure easily identified	No impression or distortion observed, bone structure easily identified	Absent
1+ Edema		Slight pitting without distortion, rapidly disappears	Barely detectable depression, immediate rebound	Mild Isolated to bilateral ankles and/or feet

2 mm

TABLE 5-5, continued

5

ASSESSMENT OF FLUID STATUS

Grade	Method 1	Method 2	Method 3
2+ Edema 4 mm	Somewhat deeper pit, distortion not easily apparent, disappears 10–25 s later	Deeper pit that takes a few seconds to rebound	Moderate Includes lower arms with hands and/or lower legs with feet/ankles
3+ Edema 6 mm	Noticeably deep pitting, entire extremity looks full, swollen; indentation can last longer than 1 min	Pit even more pronounced, taking about 10–12 s to rebound	Severe Generalized bilateral pitting edema, inclusive of upper and lower extremities and face
4+ Edema 8 mm	Very deep pitting, extremity is grossly misshapen, indentation lasts 2–5 min	Very deep, 8-mm pit taking longer than 20 s to rebound	Not applicable

TIPS

TABLE 5-6. EVALUATION OF FLUID ACCUMULATION/EDEMA

	Inspection	Palpation
When to perform	At initial visit Reevaluate at routine intervals (eg, with reassessment of nutrition status or when a significant change in medical condition occurs)	At initial visit Reevaluate at routine intervals (eg, with reassessment of nutrition status or when a significant change in medical condition occurs)
Areas of concern	Use of head-to-toe procedure • Face, arms, hands • Sacral area, scrotum, vulva • Flanks, abdomen • Thighs, calves, feet	Focused evaluation of • Sacral area, flanks • Thighs, calves, feet
Special considerations	Observe body position (eg, sitting, standing, lying down), as gravity influences fluid accumulation Observe if swelling is • Generalized or localized • Unilateral or bilateral	Observe body position (eg, sitting, standing, lying down), as gravity influences fluid accumulation Observe if swelling is • Generalized or localized • Unilateral or bilateral • Pitting or brawny

Dehydration and Hypovolemia

Although dehydration and hypovolemia are not characteristics used to determine whether malnutrition is present,[2] it is important to understand that patients with these conditions will clinically present with a falsely low weight. This can skew the final malnutrition diagnosis by overestimating the perceived weight loss amount. The etiologies of dehydration and volume depletion are multifaceted and beyond the scope of this discussion.[14] It can be very difficult to evaluate dehydration/hypovolemia, even for experienced practitioners. The clinical exam tends to be insensitive and nonspecific [14,28] and is not dependent on a single indictor.[14,28] Observations from a physical exam, in conjunction with assessment of weight, vital signs, and laboratory values, will lead to proper evaluation of hydration (Figure 5-1 and Table 5-7).[14]

FIGURE 5-1. CLINICAL SYMPTOMS OF DEHYDRATION[14,28]

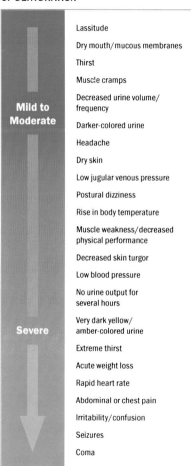

Mild to Moderate

Lassitude

Dry mouth/mucous membranes

Thirst

Muscle cramps

Decreased urine volume/ frequency

Darker-colored urine

Headache

Dry skin

Low jugular venous pressure

Postural dizziness

Rise in body temperature

Muscle weakness/decreased physical performance

Decreased skin turgor

Low blood pressure

No urine output for several hours

Very dark yellow/ amber-colored urine

Extreme thirst

Acute weight loss

Rapid heart rate

Abdominal or chest pain

Irritability/confusion

Seizures

Coma

Severe

TABLE 5-7. LABORATORY VALUES AND VITAL SIGNS ASSOCIATED WITH DEHYDRATION[14]

Laboratory/Vital Sign	Result	Additional Considerations
Serum sodium	↑ Hypernatremia ↓ Hyponatremia	In cases of water loss In cases of water and sodium loss
Serum potassium	↑ Hyperkalemia ↓ Hypokalemia	In cases of water loss but potassium retention (eg, renal failure) In cases of significant GI or urine losses
Plasma osmolality	↑	N/A
BUN/Cr ratio	↑	Often >20:1
Hematocrit	↑	Due to reduction in plasma volume
Albumin	↑ Hyperalbuminemia	Due to reduction in plasma volume
Metabolic acidosis	Present/not present	In cases of loss of bicarbonate (eg, GI losses via diarrhea or high fistula/ ostomy output)
Metabolic alkalosis	Present/not present	In cases of hydrogen ion loss (eg, diuretics, significant emesis, or nasogastric tube suctioning)
Urine sodium concentration	↓	In cases of hypovolemia (unless accompanied by salt-wasting state)
Blood pressure	↓ Bradycardia	Postural signs initially, then persistent despite posture as dehydration worsens
Heart rate	Tachycardia	N/A

BUN, blood urea nitrogen; Cr, creatinine; GI, gastrointestinal; N/A, not applicable.

TABLE 5-8. AREAS OF FOCUS TO EVALUATE FOR DEHYDRATION[14,28]

Area	Technique	Normal	Dehydrated
Mouth — Lips, Gums, Tongue 	Visual inspection (penlight is useful)	Will appear moist	Lack of saliva pooling, thick-appearing saliva, dry mucous membranes, fissured tongue, lips/tongue sticking together, cracked lips, complaints of thirst
Eyes 	Visual inspection (penlight is useful)	Membranes will appear moist	Stinging or burning feeling, membranes look dry, redness, watery eyes
Skin[a] 	Turgor assessment: Pinch skin for a few seconds on the back of the hand, forearm, or sternum	After letting go, skin should quickly return to its original position	After letting go, skin slowly returns to the original position

TABLE 5-8, continued

Area	Technique	Normal	Dehydrated
Nails			
	With patient's hand at a level above the heart, apply pressure to the nail bed until it turns white (indicates blood was forced from tissue), and then remove pressure	Blood should return, causing nail bed to turn pink within 2 s after pressure is relieved	Refill times longer than 2 s could indicate dehydration (also: shock, peripheral vascular disease, hypothermia)

ªThis is a reliable indicator in younger patients, but in patients with obesity or who are >55–60 years old, turgor may not be accurate; skin elasticity is best preserved on sternum or inner aspect of thigh.[14]

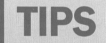

Infants, young children, athletes, elderly people, and individuals who are cognitively impaired are at higher risk of dehydration. Additional conditions that increase risk of dehydration include[14,28]

- Excessive diarrhea or vomiting
- Profuse sweating
- Gastrointestinal hemorrhage
- Gastrointestinal losses via fistulae, ostomies, or external drainage
- Polyuria (ie, diabetes insipidus, diuretics use)

- Fevers
- Burns
- Exposure to warm environments
- Prolonged exercise/strenuous activity

6

Functional
Status

OVERVIEW

Reduced muscle strength is a noted predictor of survival during critical illness.[7] The decline in strength and physical performance resulting from loss of muscle and function are detectable in advanced malnutrition syndromes (Table 6-1).[3] Decreased grip strength is noted as a reliable predictor of increased length of hospital stays, poor quality and quantity of life, and increased risk of mortality.[29] Nutrient deficiencies and malfunctioning organ systems contribute to the decline in functional status. Inflammation and/or infection can increase the risk for, or worsen, a malnutrition condition with a decreased response to nutrition interventions and a potential increase in mortality.[3] The combination of immobility, inflammation, inadequate feeding,[15] and insulin resistance is a pro-inflammatory process, and protein turnover and drugs may have a synergistic impact on muscle catabolism.[7]

TABLE 6-1. REDUCED GRIP STRENGTH AS A SUPPORTIVE CLINICAL CHARACTERISTIC FOR MALNUTRITION[2]

Etiology of Malnutrition	Moderate (Nonsevere)	Severe
Acute illness/injury	Not applicable	Measurably reduced
Chronic illness	Not applicable	Measurably reduced
Social/environmental circumstance	Not applicable	Measurably reduced

Measuring Functional Status

The use of a handgrip dynamometer as a measurement of muscle strength is a validated approach for determining an individual's functional status.[3,30,31] The Jamar dynamometer is the validated device for measuring handgrip strength.[32] Impaired grip strength may help identify patients at risk for increased postoperative complications, longer hospitalizations, rehospitalization, and decreased physical status. Findings from handgrip dynamometry are a relevant marker of functional status and are useful in the assessment of nutrition status.[31]

In some clinical settings, use of the dynamometer may not be available or practical.[31] Identifying other potential performance measures to aid in the evaluation of functional status may also be useful as they become accepted or are validated.[2] As previously noted, suggestions for using gait speed and chair standing tests as potential options of functional measurements are being discussed.[15]

Quality-of-life tools that also consider functional ability, such as the Katz Index of Independence in Activities of Daily Living, Lawton Instrumental Activities of Daily Living, Karnofsky Performance Scale Index, and the Eastern Cooperative Oncology Group Scale of Performance Status may provide supplementary information on an individual's performance status.[31]

Validated nutrition assessment tools that include functional status measures include the Subjective Global Assessment (SGA),[6] Dialysis Malnutrition Score,[33,34] and Patient-Generated SGA.[35]

Techniques for Using a Handgrip Dynamometer

The preferred protocol is the American Society of Hand Therapists' method.[32] This "gold standard" technique utilizes rapid exchange of 3 alternating hand sequential measurements. Rapid exchange allows for recovery from muscle fatigue and prevents patients from malingering or using submaximal effort. A total of 6 readings should be performed during the test so that a mean can be calculated for each hand. This result can then be compared with the standard normal reference tables provided by the dynamometer manufacturer to determine upper-extremity strength as a proxy for overall body strength.

Steps

1. Seat patient in standardized position (Figure 6-1).

   a. In an armchair: sitting upright with arms unsupported

   b. In a bed: sitting upright at side of bed or in bed with legs out straight (at 90° angle to upper body)

   c. Shoulders are relaxed, elbow is at right angle, and wrist is not bent

2. Allow patient to rest for 15 seconds between trials.

3. Continue to test (making sure to alternate hands each time) and record values until 3 measures have been obtained for each hand.

4. Calculate the sum of the 3 values on each side. Divide by 3 to get the mean (average).

5. Compare this result to the manufacturer's chart that is included with the dynamometer.

FIGURE 6-1. HANDGRIP DYNAMOMETER POSITION

✔ CORRECT

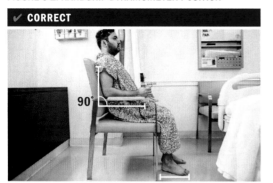

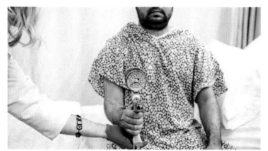

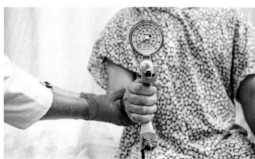

✘ INCORRECT

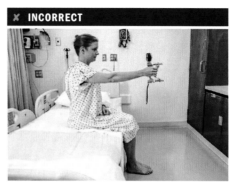

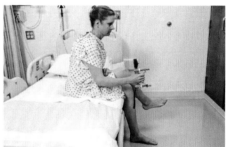

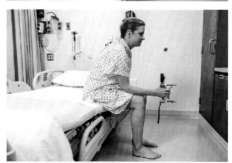

7

Micronutrient Status

OVERVIEW

Although not included as 1 of the Academy of Nutrition and Dietetics (Academy)/American Society for Parenteral and Enteral Nutrition (ASPEN) characteristics to diagnose malnutrition, micronutrient deficiencies can provide supporting evidence for the malnutrition diagnosis.[36] Determining micronutrient deficiencies or excesses, and detecting clues to macronutrient deficiency by physical exam, further provides insight into nutrient ingestion, digestion, absorption, and metabolism. Those who possess the greatest risk factors for micronutrient deficiencies are those with chronic conditions, such as malabsorptive conditions, pancreatic insufficiency, and/or end-stage renal disease, and those who have restricted diets or lack of access to food.[37] Micronutrient deficiencies and excesses may be readily seen in the skin, nails, hair, eyes, and orofacial area. It is also important to ascertain awareness of differential diagnosis for physical signs that may occur because of nonnutrition factors.[37]

Skin

Skin, the largest organ of the human body, accounts for 16% of total body weight and can often reveal vitamin and mineral deficiencies (Table 7-1).[38,39] Micronutrient abnormalities may appear rapidly because of skin-cell turnover every 10–30 days.[40]

TABLE 7-1. PHYSICAL ASSESSMENT OF MICRONUTRIENTS: SKIN[39-42]

Physical Sign	Possible Nutrient Finding	Possible Nonnutrient Causes
Petechiae (small hemorrhagic spots on skin)	Vitamin K, E, and/or C deficiency	Hematologic disorder Liver disease Anticoagulant overdose
Dermatitis (swollen, reddened skin that may blister or ooze)	Zinc deficiency Essential fatty acid deficiency	Dermatitis Allergic or medication-related rashes Psoriasis
Pellagrous dermatosis (hyperpigmentation of areas exposed to sunlight/trauma)	Niacin deficiency Tryptophan deficiency	Burns Addison's disease Psoriasis
Flaky paint dermatitis (bilateral "peeling paint"–looking skin of areas usually not exposed to sunlight)	Protein-calorie deficiency	Environmental factors

TABLE 7-1, continued

MICRONUTRIENT STATUS

Physical Sign	Possible Nutrient Finding	Possible Nonnutrient Causes
Xerosis (dry, scaly, flaky skin)	Dehydration Essential fatty acid deficiency Vitamin A deficiency	Environmental factors Hygiene factors
Poor pallor (pale skin color)	Iron deficiency Folate deficiency Vitamin B_{12} deficiency	Low-volume, low-perfusion states
Nonhealing wounds	Zinc deficiency Ascorbic acid deficiency Protein deficiency	Cellulitis

This table is not intended to be a complete list of nutrition or nonnutrition causes for presenting physical signs and symptoms.

TIPS

- Skin integrity and elasticity are altered by sun/ultraviolet light, age, and hydration.[41]

- Allergies and medications may cause rashes; nutrition abnormalities may cause pigment changes and rashes.[40,42]

Nails

Nail growth is determined by the matrix cells, with cell turnover varying by digit location or by hereditary circumstances. On average, thumbnail growth is 0.10–0.12 mm/day. Nail changes can be a result of nutrition deficiencies as well as systemic diseases. Keratin, the fibrous protein of which the nail is composed, should be firmly adhered to the nail bed, feel smooth, and appear uniformly thick and symmetrical.[43] Healthy nails are translucent with a pink hue, are flat or slightly convex, and have a base angle equal to 160°. Several nail-nutrient findings are depicted in Table 7-2.

TABLE 7-2. PHYSICAL ASSESSMENT OF MICRONUTRIENTS: NAILS[37,39-42]

	Physical Sign	Possible Nutrient Finding	Possible Nonnutrient Causes
	Koilonychia (spoon-shaped nails)	Iron deficiency, with or without anemia	Hereditary Infection Diabetes Hypothyroidism Acromegaly Hematologic conditions Trauma Carpal tunnel syndrome
	Beau's/transverse line (horizontal grooves)	Protein inadequacy Hypercalcemia	Trauma Coronary occlusion Skin disease Transient illness

TABLE 7-2, continued

Physical Sign		Possible Nutrient Finding	Possible Nonnutrient Causes
	Poor blanching of nails (pale nail bed)	Vitamin A and vitamin C deficiency	Poor circulation
	Splinter hemorrhages	Scurvy or hemochromatosis	Septicemia Trauma Hemodialysis
	Poor nail-plate health (whitened areas on nail beds)	Selenium deficiency	Trauma Environmental factors

TABLE 7-2, continued

Physical Sign	Possible Nutrient Finding	Possible Nonnutrient Causes
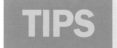 **Flaky nails**	Hypomagnesaemia Biotin deficiency Essential fatty acid deficiency	Trauma Environmental factors
Clubbing (nail plate exceeding 180°)	None	Respiratory disorder Cardiovascular disease Cirrhosis Colitis

This table is not intended to be a complete list of nutrition or nonnutrition causes for presenting physical signs and symptoms.

TIPS

- To assess capillary refill, gently squeeze the nail between the thumb and forefinger to palpate; if bleeding occurs, may indicate general malnutrition.

- Lackluster or dull appearance of nail plate may indicate protein deficiency, but may also be indicative of infection or systemic lupus erythematous.

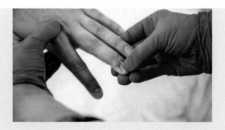

Hair

Hair change and growth (0.3 mm/day of growth) is similar to rapid nail cell turnover and the skin's ability to reflect changes in micronutrient status (Table 7-3). Healthy hair is shiny, smooth, resilient, and not easily plucked.[41] Poor hair quality can be associated with protein, zinc, essential fatty acid, and biotin deficiencies.

TABLE 7-3. PHYSICAL ASSESSMENT OF MICRONUTRIENTS: HAIR[39-42,44]

Physical Sign		Possible Nutrient Finding	Possible Nonnutrient Causes
	Alopecia (hair thinning or loss)	Protein, zinc, and/or biotin deficiency diffuse loss (including eyebrows): essential fatty acids or selenium deficiency	Male-pattern baldness Hypopituitarism Hypothyroidism Cancer treatment Chemical alteration Infection Psoriasis Cushing's disease Medication
	Lightened hair color	Copper deficiency Selenium deficiency Protein deficiency	Chemical alteration

TABLE 7-3, continued

Physical Sign	Possible Nutrient Finding	Possible Nonnutrient Causes
Corkscrew hair (located on arms)	Copper deficiency, follicular hyperkeratosis from scurvy in elderly people[36]	Chemical alteration

This table is not intended to be a complete list of nutrition or nonnutrition causes for presenting physical signs and symptoms.

TIPS

- Lackluster or dull hair may indicate iron, protein, and/or zinc deficiency; consider chemical treatment. Ask the patient if their hair has been colored or altered.

- Palpate hair to determine if hair is resilient and not easily plucked. Ask the patient if they are noticing hair falling out more often. Take note of any hair on their pillow or clothing.

Orofacial

Examination of the eyes, face, lips, and oral cavity may reveal micronutrient deficiencies and can correlate with findings of the skin, nails, hair, and diet history (Table 7-4). For example, vitamin A deficiency may manifest as night blindness and may also present as Bitot's spots on the eye and keratomalacia.[40] The oral mucosa's cell turnover is <1 week; therefore, nutrient deficiencies can be detected quickly and routine monitoring can be useful for assessing the effectiveness of ones' medical nutrition therapy.[45] The Academy supports the collaboration between dietetic and dental professionals for disease prevention and nutrition and dental intervention of the oral cavity.[46]

TABLE 7-4. PHYSICAL ASSESSMENT OF MICRONUTRIENTS: OROFACIAL[36,39-42,46]

Physical Sign		Possible Nutrient Finding	Possible Nonnutrient Causes
	Nasolabial seborrhea (scaling around nostrils)	Vitamin B_2, B_3, and/or B_6 deficiency	Tuberous sclerosis
	Bitot's spot (gray spongy spot on white of the eye)	Vitamin A deficiency	Pinguecula (elderly people) Gaucher disease (hereditary) Pterygium

TABLE 7-4, continued

Physical Sign		Possible Nutrient Finding	Possible Nonnutrient Causes
	Keratomalacia (hazy cornea)	Vitamin A deficiency	Hyperthyroidism
	Pale conjunctivae	Iron deficiency Folate deficiency Vitamin B_{12} deficiency	Low cardiac-output states
	Cheilosis	Vitamin B_2, B_3, and/or B_6 deficiency Iron deficiency	Environmental Herpes
	Angular stomatitis (bilateral cracks and redness of lips)	Vitamin B_2, B_3, and/or B_6 deficiency Iron deficiency	Irritation from ill-fitting dentures Herpes Chapping from harsh climate Infectious disease

TABLE 7-4, continued

Physical Sign		Possible Nutrient Finding	Possible Nonnutrient Causes
	Spongy, bloody gums	Vitamin C deficiency	Gingivitis (due to poor hygiene, malocclusion, dental caries) Amyloidosis Acute myeloid leukemia Drugs Periodontal disease
	Mouth lesions	Zinc deficiency	Trauma Graft-vs-host disease Cancer treatment
	Pale gum color	Iron deficiency	Low flow state
	Glossitis (inflammation of tongue, magenta in color)	Vitamin B_2, B_3, B_6, and/or B_{12} deficiency Folate deficiency Iron deficiency (severe)	Crohn's disease Uremia Infection Malignancy Anticancer therapy Trauma

TABLE 7-4, continued

Physical Sign		Possible Nutrient Finding	Possible Nonnutrient Causes
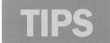	Enlarged parotid (bilateral)	Protein inadequacy	Bulimia, excessive vomiting, mumps, portal cirrhosis, Sjogren's syndrome (usually females), allergic or inflammatory process, neoplasm, sarcoidosis, sialolithiasis
	Enlarged thyroid	Iodine deficiency	Mumps, allergy or inflammatory process, Graves' disease, malignancy, thyroglossal duct cyst, thyroiditis, bronchial cleft cysts, and tumors

This table is not intended to be a complete list of nutrition or nonnutrition causes for presenting physical signs and symptoms.

TIPS

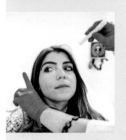

EYES

- Probe patient and ask if they have difficulty seeing and/or abnormal eye dryness that may indicate a vitamin A deficiency (eye dryness may also be from general environmental irritation).

- Direct patient to look side to side to see entire eye.

- Hold up your index finger and instruct the patient to follow your finger with their eye. As you move your finger to the right or left, shine a penlight onto the patient's sclera. Try not to shine the light directly into the patient's pupil.

ORAL CAVITY [46]

- Direct patient to move tongue from side to side and lift tongue.

- Direct patient to stick out tongue.

- May also want to observe the patient swallowing or inquire about their ability to swallow.

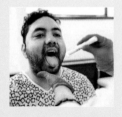

Ask these questions to distinguish between nonnutrient cause and nutrient cause:

1. Do you have any changes in taste?

2. Do you have any burning sensations in your mouth?

3. Do you have any mouth pain or notice gum bleeding?

Appendix 1

NUTRITION-FOCUSED PHYSICAL EXAM CHECKLIST

NUTRITION-FOCUSED PHYSICAL EXAM CHECKLIST

Region	Location	Task	Check if Performed
Skin	All applicable	Throughout the entire examination, the registered dietitian observes the skin for the following: • dermatitis • scaliness • poor wound healing • rashes • dryness • poor turgor • petechiae • presence of • ecchymosis pressure ulcers	
Head	Hair	Touch and observe for the following: • thinness • brittleness • dullness • patchy growth • dryness • easily pluckable	
	ᵃTemple	Standing directly in front of patient, palpate temporalis muscles. Check for fullness and firmness. Observe for depression, hollowing.	
	Mouth	Have patient open mouth and shine penlight into oral cavity. Next, have patient stick out tongue. Observe for the following: • Mucosa: pallor, dryness, decreased salivary flow, ulcerations (mucositis) • Tongue: magenta or beefy red color; smooth, slick appearance (glossitis)	
	Teeth	Observe for tooth decay, missing teeth.	
	Gums	Observe for sponginess, bleeding; swollen, red, receding gums.	
	ᵃEyes	Orbital pads: While standing directly in front of patient, gently palpate area below eyes. Observe for darkness, hollowness, and/or loose skin.	
		Observe for cracked or reddened corners of eyes, foamy (Bitot's spots) areas on sclera; dull, dry, or rough sclera; dull, milky, opaque cornea.	

Region	Location	Task	Check if Performed
Upper body	Chest	Have patient assume upright posture and gently palpate pectoralis muscles below/along clavicles for fullness and firmness. Observe for prominence of clavicles.	
	Shoulders[a]	Palpate deltoid muscles for fullness and firmness. Observe for squaring of shoulders.	
	Back	Have patient sit forward and palpate trapezius and/or latissimus dorsi muscles for fullness and firmness. Observe for prominence of scapula, spine, and ribs.	
	Midaxillary line	Have patient lift arm, and palpate ribs along midaxillary line. Observe for prominence of ribs and iliac crest.	
	Triceps skinfold[a]	Have patient bend arm at 90° angle with upper arm perpendicular to body; if the patient is unable to cooperate, bend elbow at 90° and place forearm horizontally across body if possible; grasp upper arm midway between shoulder and elbow with palm and fingers and gradually pull skin away from arm with fingers while wiggling slightly to separate fat from muscle.	
	Hands[a]	Have patient make "OK" sign with thumb and first finger and while palpating interosseous muscle between thumb and first finger and the interosseous muscles between remaining fingers. Check for fullness and firmness.	
		Observe for depression.	
		Observe for missing, misshapen (spoon-shaped), or splintered fingernails and transverse ridging, discoloration, dullness, lackluster appearance, and mottling of nails.	
Lower body	Thighs[a]	Palpate for fullness and firmness. Observe for roundness/fullness of muscle and prominence of patella.	
	Calves[a]	Have patient bend knees at 90° angle if possible. Grasp calves with palm and fingers to determine fullness and firmness. Observe for roundness.	
	Lower legs/feet[a]	Observe for swelling of feet. Note any asymmetry between left and right. Press top of each foot with thumb or finger with moderate pressure for several seconds, release, and observe for depth of depression and refill time. Note any difference in left vs. right. Repeat on lower legs.	

[a] Bilateral examination should be performed.

Appendix 2

RECOMMENDED DOCUMENTATION PRACTICES FOR
SUCCESSFUL CODING OF MALNUTRITION

RECOMMENDED DOCUMENTATION PRACTICES FOR SUCCESSFUL CODING OF MALNUTRITION[2,47]

Ensure that a policy, approved by medical staff, exists at your institution stating the method that will be used to identify malnutrition.

Educate healthcare providers, coders, and documentation specialists on this method to improve awareness of malnutrition, create understanding of the method, provide transparency across disciplines, and encourage agreement among the medical team. Coders and documentation specialists can then make sure *ICD-10* codes are applied properly:

- E43   Unspecified severe protein-calorie malnutrition
- E44.0 Moderate protein-calorie malnutrition

Work with the information technology department, coders, and documentation specialists to develop consistent and specific language that efficiently and accurately captures the malnutrition diagnosis. This should include the ability to readily identify the following:

- The presence and severity of malnutrition based on a specific etiologic framework
- Evidence for each of the malnutrition characteristics
- A plan of care to treat malnutrition
- The manner in which the plan will be monitored and evaluated

Ensure dietitians are competent in consistently assessing and interpreting all characteristics of malnutrition, including the NFPE.

Dietitians provide *recommendations* regarding the degree of malnutrition on the basis of a specified etiology that are supported with evidence of applicable characteristics in the medical record.

Dos

- Confirm that the characteristics align with the chosen etiology.
- Ensure that the minimum threshold is met (within the chosen etiology) to define the severity of malnutrition.

Don'ts

- Document contradictions within the same entry without further clarification.
- Recommend a malnutrition diagnosis if you don't have adequate information.

Dos

- Document NFPE results in a manner that is clear and specific.

- Rule out causes of muscle/fat losses from nonnutrition sources; the NFPE needs to substantiate other evidence in the medical chart.

- Aim to evaluate as many muscle and fat areas as possible to determine losses related to malnutrition. No minimal requirements exist regarding the number of areas that need to be observed; this is a clinical decision based on individual cases.

- Verify subjective data with more objective evidence; use clinical judgment to understand the entire picture of an individual case.

- Be accurate and thorough but concise. It is okay to say "unable to identify" malnutrition and then reevaluate at a later date.

Don'ts

- Document NFPE results or other characteristics in a vague or confusing manner.

- Make assumptions about observations during the NFPE.

- "Diagnose" malnutrition; this must be a recommendation provided to a physician or licensed independent practitioner.

- Provide documentation that is lengthy, repetitive, or incomplete.

- State "unable to identify" malnutrition without having a consistent plan for reevaluation.

Dietitians communicate the degree of malnutrition to the primary care providers in a manner that is most effective for your institution.
If the physician or licensed independent practitioner agrees with recommendations, this is documented in the patient's medical-record note.
Documentation by the dietitian should also include an intervention with an established monitoring and evaluation plan.

ICD-10, *International Classification of Diseases, Tenth Revision;* NFPE, nutrition-focused physical exam.

EXAMPLE OF ELECTRONIC-MEDICAL-RECORD DOCUMENTATION[2]

Recommended diagnosis (choose 1):

No malnutrition · Moderate protein-calorie malnutrition
Severe protein-calorie malnutrition · Unable to determine

In the context of (choose 1):

Acute injury/illness · Chronic illness · Social/environmental

Based on (choose all that apply):

Weight loss · Inadequate energy intakes · Muscle loss
Fluid accumulation · Functional decline · Fat loss

Intervention/treatment plan (free text area and/or selection of frequently used interventions):

_____

Monitoring & evaluation (free text area and/or selection of frequently used monitors):

_____
_____

History of present illness (free text area for relevant details):

_____

Diet order/supplements (auto-populated):

Nutrition intakes (compared to estimated energy needs):			
>75%	<75%	≤50%	Unable to determine
Free text area for additional details:			

Over:			
>7 days	≥5 days	≥1 month	≥3 months

Nutrition intake history: (free text area for relevant details)

_____

GI symptoms: (free text area for relevant details)

Anthropometrics: (some portions auto-populated)

Height: _____ Current Weight: _____ Usual Body Weight: _____ Body Mass Index: _____

Weight changes (choose 1)

1%–2% in 1 week	5% in 1 month	7.5% in 3 months	10% in 6 months	20% in 12 months
>2% in 1 week	>5% in 1 month	>7.5% in 3 months	>10% in 6 months	>20% in 12 months
None	Unable to determine			

Physical exam:

Muscle loss (choose 1)

None	Mild	Moderate	Severe	Unable to determine

Fat loss (choose 1)

None	Mild	Moderate	Severe	Unable to determine

Fluid accumulation

Location:	Upper extremities	Lower extremities	Generalized	Ascites
None	Mild	Moderate	Severe	Unable to determine
None	1+	2+	3-4+	Unable to determine

Functional capacity (choose 1)

Normal	Regressed	Handgrip measurably reduced	Not related to nutrition status

Markers of inflammation (choose all that apply)

Hypoalbuminemia	Elevated CRP	Acute post-op	Sepsis
Fevers	Tachycardia	Low pre-albumin	Hyperglycemia

Signature plate:

Clinician name: _____ Credentials: _____

Contact information: _____

CRP, C-reactive protein; post-op, postoperative.

References

1. Brantley SL, Russell MK, Mogensen KM, et al. American Society for Parenteral and Enteral Nutrition and Academy of Nutrition and Dietetics revised 2014 standards of practice and standards of professional performance for registered dietitian nutritionists (competent, proficient, and expert) in nutrition support. *J Acad Nutr Diet.* 2014;114(12):2001–2008, e37.

2. White JV, Guenter P, Jensen G, et al. Consensus statement: Academy of Nutrition and Dietetics and American Society for Parenteral and Enteral Nutrition: characteristics recommended for the identification and documentation of adult malnutrition (undernutrition) [erratum in *JPEN J Parenter Enteral Nutr.* 2017;41(3):520]. *JPEN J Parenter Enteral Nutr.* 2012;36(3):275–283.

3. Jensen G, Hsiao PY, Wheeler D. Adult nutrition assessment tutorial. *JPEN J Parenter Enteral Nutr.* 2012;36(3):267–274.

4. Jevenn A, Galang M, Hipskind P, Bury C. Malnutrition screening and assessment. In: Mueller CM, ed. *ASPEN Adult Nutrition Support Core Curriculum.* 3rd ed. American Society for Parenteral and Enteral Nutrition; 2017:186–209

5. Secker DJ, Jeejeebhoy KN. How to perform subjective global nutritional assessment in children. *J Acad Nutr Diet.* 2012(3);112:424–431.

6. Detsky AS, McLaughlin JR, Baker JP, et al. What is subjective global assessment of nutritional status? *JPEN J Parenter Enteral Nutr.* 1987;11(1):8–13.

7. Puthucheary Z, Montgomery H, Moxham J, Harridge S, Hart N. Structure to function: muscle failure in critically ill patients. *J Physiol.* 2010;588(Pt 23):4641–4648.

8. Standards for privacy of individually identifiable health information: final privacy rule preamble. US Department of Health & Human Services. Updated December 28, 2000. Accessed August 15, 2020. https://aspe.hhs.gov/report/standards-privacy-individually-identifiable-health-information-final-privacy-rule-preamble

9. Fischer M, Jevenn A, Hipskind P. Evaluation for muscle and fat loss as diagnostic criteria for malnutrition. *Nutr Clin Pract.* 2015;30(2):243–248.

10. Siegel JD, Rhinehart E, Jackson M, Chiarello L, Healthcare Infection Control Practices Advisory Committee. Guideline for isolation precautions: preventing transmission of infectious agents in healthcare settings (2007). Centers for Disease Control and Prevention. Updated July 2019. Accessed August 15, 2020. https://www.cdc.gov/infectioncontrol/guidelines/isolation/index.html

11. Smith CC. Clinical manifestations and evaluation of edema in adults. In: Post TW, ed. *UpToDate.* UpToDate; 2019. Accessed August 5, 2020. https://www.uptodate.com

12. Edema grading. Med-Health.net. Accessed August 1, 2020. https://www.med-health.net/edema-grading.html

13. Dugdale DC. Capillary nail refill test. MedlinePlus. Updated April 26, 2019. Accessed August 1, 2020. https://medlineplus.gov/ency/article/003394.htm

14. Part 17: edema. In: Stern SDC, Cifu AS, Altkorn D, eds. *Symptom to Diagnosis: An Evidence-Based Guide.* 4th ed. McGraw-Hill Educational; 2020. Accessed August 1, 2020. https://accessmedicine.mhmedical.com/book.aspx?bookid=2715

15. Cederholm T, Barazzoni R, Austin P, et al. ESPEN guidelines on definitions and terminology of clinical nutrition. *Clin Nutr.* 2017;36(1):49–64.

16. Malone A, Hamilton C. The Academy of Nutrition and Dietetics/The American Society for Parenteral and Enteral Nutrition consensus malnutrition characteristics: application in practice. *Nutr Clin Pract.* 2013(6);28:639–650.

17. Kushner I, Samols D, Magrey M. A Unifying biologic explanation for "high-sensitivity" C-reactive protein and "low-grade" inflammation. *Arthritis Care Res.* 2010;62(4):442–446.

18. Pagana KD, Pagana TJ, Pagana TN. *Mosby's Diagnostic and Laboratory Test Reference.* 12th ed. Elsevier; 2015.

19. Jensen GL. Malnutrition and inflammation—"burning down the house": inflammation as an adaptive physiologic response versus self-destruction? *JPEN J Parenter Enteral Nutr.* 2015;39(1):56–62.

20. Nicolo M, Compher CW, Still C, Huseini M, Dayto S, Jensen GL. Feasibility of accessing data in hospitalized patients to support diagnosis of malnutrition by the Academy–A.S.P.E.N. malnutrition consensus recommended clinical characteristics. *JPEN J Parenter Enteral Nutr.* 2014;38(8):954–959.

21. Puthucheary ZA, Rawal J, McPhail M, et al. Acute skeletal muscle wasting in critical illness. *JAMA.* 2013;310(15):1591–1600.

22. Prado CM, Heymsfield SB. Lean tissue imaging: a new era for nutritional assessment and intervention. *JPEN J Parenter Enteral Nutr.* 2014;38(8):940–53.

23. Jensen GL, Cederholm T, Correia MI, et al. GLIM criteria for the diagnosis of malnutrition: a consensus report from the global clinical nutrition community. *JPEN J Parenter Enteral Nutr.* 2019;43(1):32–40.

24. Coltman A, Peterson S, Roehl K, et al. Use of 3 tools to assess nutrition risk in the intensive care unit. *JPEN J Parenter Enteral Nutr.* 2015;39(1):28–33.

25. Keys A. Caloric undernutrition and starvation, with notes on protein deficiency. *J Am Med Assoc.* 1948;138(7):500–511.

26. Rosenthal LD, Cumbler E. Evaluation of peripheral edema. Epocrates. Updated April 14, 2020. Accessed August 1, 2020. https://online.epocrates.com/diseases/609/Evaluation-of-peripheral-edema

27. Braunwald E, Loscalzo J. Chapter 37: edema. In: Jameson LJ, Fauci AS, Kasper DL, Hauser SL, Longo DL, Loscalzo J, eds. *Harrison's Principles of Internal Medicine.* 20th ed. McGraw Medical; 2018. Accessed online August 1, 2020. https://accessmedicine.mhmedical.com/content.aspx?bookid=2129&sectionid=192012582

28. Jéquier E, Constant F. Water as an essential nutrient: the physiological basis of hydration. *Eur J Clin Nutr.* 2010;64(2):115–123.

29. Cruz-Jentoft AJ, Bahat G, Bauer J, et al. Sarcopenia: revised European consensus on definition and diagnosis. *Age Ageing.* 2019;48(1):16–31.

30. Mueller C, McClave S, Kuhn JM. *The A.S.P.E.N. Adult Nutrition Support Core Curriculum.* 2nd ed. American Society for Parenteral and Enteral Nutrition; 2012.

31. Russell MK. Functional assessment of nutrition status. *Nutr Clin Pract*. 2015;30(2):211–218.

32. Schectman O, Sindhu BS. Grip assessment. In: MacDermid J, ed. *Clinical Assessment Recommendations*. 3rd ed. American Society of Hand Therapists; 2015:1–8 and Online Companion (1–20). http://www.asht.org

33. Zadeh K, Kleiner M, Dunne E, Lee GH, Luft FC. A modified quantitative subjective global assessment of nutrition for dialysis patients. *Nephrol Dial Transplant*. 1999;14(7):1732–1738.

34. Steiber AL, Kalantar-Zadeh K, Secker D, McCarthy M, Sehgal A, McCann L. Subjective global assessment in chronic kidney disease: a review. *J Ren Nutr*. 2004;14(4):191–200.

35. Capra S, Ferguson M. Use of the scored Patient-Generated Subjective Global Assessment (PG-SGA) as a nutrition assessment tool in patients with cancer. *Eur J Clin Nutr*. 2002;56(8):779–785.

36. Hammond KA. The nutritional dimension of physical assessment. *Nutrition*. 1999;15(5):411–419.

37. DiBaise M. Tarleton S. Hair, nails, and skin: differentiating cutaneous manifestations of micronutrient deficiency. *Nutr Clin Pract*. 2019;34(4):490–503.

38. Bickley LS. *Bates' Guide to Physical Examination and History Taking*. 10th ed. Wolters Kluwer/Lippincott Williams & Wilkins; 2009.

39. Hammond KA, Hillhouse J. *Nutrition-Focused Physical Assessment Skills for Dietitians: Study Guide*. 2nd ed. American Dietetic Association; 2000.

40. Hammond K. History and physical examination. In: Matarese LE, Gottschlich MM, eds. *Contemporary Nutrition Support Practice: A Clinical Guide*. 2nd ed. Elsevier Science; 2002:14–25.

41. Seidel HM, Stewart RW, Ball JE, Flynn JA, Solomon BS. *Mosby's Guide to Physical Examination*. 7th ed. Elsevier; 2011.

42. Morrison SG. Clinical nutrition physical examination. *Support Line*. 1997;19(2):16–18.

43. Cashman MW, Sloan SB. Nutrition and nail disease. *Clin Dermatol*. 2010;28(4):420-425.

44. Goldberg LJ, Lenzy Y. Nutrition and hair. *Clin Dermatol*. 2010;28(4):412–419.

45. Radler DR, Lister T. Nutrition deficiencies associated with nutrition focused physical findings of the oral cavity. *Nutr Clin Pract*. 2013;28(6):710–721.

46. Tougher-Decker R, Mobley C. Position of the academy of nutrition and dietetics: oral health and nutrition. *J Acad Nutr Diet*. 2013;113(5):693–701.

47. Doley J, Phillips W. Coding for malnutrition in the hospital: does it change reimbursement? *Nutr Clin Pract*. 2019;34(6):823–831.